Peripheral Neuropathy: Nine Simple Steps To Reduce The Pain

Dean S Lewis MT

Copyright © 2014 Dean S. Lewis
All rights reserved.

ISBN: 1503359689
ISBN 13: 9781503359680
Library of Congress Control Number: 2014921173
CreateSpace Independent Publishing Platform
North Charleston, South Carolina

Contents

Foreword v
Acknowledgments vii
Introduction ix
1. How "It" Started and Getting to Know Your
   Peripheral Neuropathy 1
2. Design Your Life 7
3. Mind-set and Transmutation 13
4. Nutrition 19
5. Exercise and Massage 25
6. Spirituality, Meditation, and Yoga 33
7. Dreams and Goals 39
8. Medication, Supplementation, and Devices 43
9. Live Your Life 49
Frequently Asked Questions (FAQ) 51
Speaking with Me 55
References and Resources 57

Foreword

This book is designed to show you how I went from being in a hospital bed to learning how to use a wheelchair, using a walker, and finally walking on my own again. It is designed to encourage you to live the life you want without having peripheral neuropathy or chronic pain prevent you from doing so. I have discovered these steps through my daily life to complement the medications I was taking. Today, I don't take any medication for my peripheral neuropathy. This decision was made many years ago after consulting with my physician and weaning off my medications.

The contents of this book are for informational purposes only and should not be used for self-diagnosis or self-treatment. This information is not intended to be substituted for medical advice. Always consult a medical professional regarding your peripheral neuropathy or other medical problems.

*This book is protected by copyright laws. It should not be copied, distributed, or sold without having received prior consent from the author.

There are links in this book from which I receive compensation.

Acknowledgments

I want to thank my mom, Marcia; my dad, Ludwell; my grandma, Valda; my aunt, Colet; my sisters, Tracey-Ann and Celia; my brother, Kristopher; and my lovely wife, Tanya, for their support during this process. I also want to thank my son, Preston, for inspiring me to continue this journey. Thank you to the members of Team Kava Mastermind for encouraging me to pursue my passion of helping others. To the dearest of friends who were with me from the start and gave me rides to my doctors and physical therapy appointments, to the members of my local peripheral neuropathy group, and for those who made the purchase, thank you for your support.

Introduction

You may be saying, "Nine steps?" Some may say that is too much or too little. Even so, I have been able to live a full life, even though I have had peripheral neuropathy for close to fourteen years. I first developed peripheral neuropathy in 1998 after having multiorgan system failure. At the time, I was given so many medications, including antibiotics, steroids, insulin, and many more, to keep me alive as my body was failing by the minute. My body went through this roller coaster for over two months, and there are parts I don't even remember because I was put into an induced coma as part of saving my life. I am here, writing this book now, because those doctors did a marvelous job. I have been able to work full time, pursue my passions (which includes going to the gym—an important requirement with my neuropathy), driving in a dragster, and tandem skydiving, to name a few.

This book is for you if you experience any of the following:

- Uncontrollable pain
- Frustration
- Unhappiness
- Despair
- Depression

- Fear (losing your job, taking care of yourself, fear of the unknown)
- Feeling that no one can relate to your pain

I have experienced one or more of these more than once over the last fourteen years. However, I have triumphed. You can too!

I wrote this book to share how these nine steps have helped reduce my pain from peripheral neuropathy. I have found these steps to be relatively simple to incorporate into my daily life, and my hope is that you will find it to be the same.

My hope is that this book will help you realize how to

1. take control of your peripheral neuropathy;
2. do things you love and are able to do safely (dancing, taking walks with your loved ones, going on vacations, exercising);
3. have peace of mind;
4. have a deeper understanding of yourself with peripheral neuropathy; and
5. transform your life of pain, resentment, and frustration into a life that is rich and full.

One

How "It" Started and Getting to Know Your Peripheral Neuropathy

I discovered that I had peripheral neuropathy during the recovery process from a multiorgan system failure. Your discovery could have occurred when you found out about your diabetes, after a critical illness like myself, after a sports injury, due to an autoimmune disease, or from other situations. The newly discovered causes for peripheral neuropathy grow each day.

My journey began on a Sunday morning, July 26, when I felt weak and had to sit down. I was at church, serving as an usher. I was only 25 years old, and in great physical shape, so I was not worried. I remember having my best friend drive me home because I was still feeling weak at the end of church service. I did feel well enough to go to an anniversary celebration later that evening. I ate, talked, laughed, and played one of my favorite games, volleyball. My girlfriend at the time drove me home, and I got ready for bed. Little did I know that round two was about to start. I suddenly had such intense abdominal pain that I don't know if the words "call the ambulance" actually made it out of my mouth. My bedroom was in the basement, so no one heard me, nor could I reach for my phone to call 911 myself.

I woke up the next morning sweating and cold. I took a shower, got dressed, and asked my sister to accompany me to the doctor. I felt strong enough to drive my car the short distance to the doctor with my sister beside me. I got to the doctor, and my symptoms at the time suggested that it was a stomach issue or food poisoning. I was prescribed some medications and sent home. A week later, I went back to the doctor, but this time I had to be driven. My symptoms were worsening, and I was beginning to feel worried at this point. The doctor saw me and prescribed antibiotics. I started taking the antibiotics on a Monday, and by Thursday I had gotten much worse. I remember waking up violently from my nap on the couch. I felt like I was burning up inside. I shouted to my sisters for help and requested water. I needed water immediately—lots of water! I felt so hot that I threw the water on my face as I drank it. This was it. I told my sister to call 911.

I was rushed to the hospital, where I was admitted and a barrage of tests started. This was the beginning of August 1998. The doctors could not figure out what was wrong and why I was declining rapidly. My family did not receive the best of news, but they knew never to give up on me because I don't give up easily. The first few days were a blur for me. I remember a few visitors, but not much beyond that. I was transferred to a different hospital once I was stabilized. My situation was so bad that I was put into a medically induced coma. The hospital did a great job supporting me and keeping me alive. During this time, I remember having the craziest of dreams. They seemed so real and were worse than a scene from a sci-fi movie with monsters. I was on a cargo train that was completely dark, and these monsters were around me. However, through it all, there was someone with me, telling me it would be OK, that I should not worry. I could not see this person, but I heard the voice. I felt I was hearing family members or my guardian angel sent by God. Throughout my hospitalization, numerous organs failed. One of the last organs to fail was my heart. Thank heavens for modern technology as

I was shocked back to life. My heart started beating again, but I was unconscious and had received a tracheotomy (a hole was made in my throat so a ventilator could help me breathe). Once I awoke, my heart rate was high—in the 130s. The medical staff got my heart rate at a more stable level, but I was not out of the woods yet. Over the next few weeks, it seemed my body was beginning to heal. I had been in the hospital for two months.

I was transferred from the intensive care unit (ICU) to a step-down unit. I had a routine to follow each day. For a few hours each day, the nurse would put in a comfortable chair where I would sit, count cars, and look out for the ferry making its usual trip. I still could not talk, and my fingers were not strong enough to write. This was part of my rehabilitation, and to get me out of the bed, as laying for too long can create skin breakdown. I began taking inventory of my body to see what was working. I could hardly move any of my limbs, and my jaw felt like it was wired shut. I decided not to panic, as I studied clinical laboratory sciences, so I was familiar with the human body. I decided to help my body along. I started visualizing doing daily activities like waking up, brushing my teeth, and so forth. One of my favorites was visualizing driving my manual transmission car. I was feeling good.

I can remember clearly in October of 1998 when I was assisted to a seating position on my hospital bed by a nursing assistant and felt the one of the worst pains I have ever felt. It felt as if I had just stepped in a large nest of red ants that bite the living daylights out of you. Only it felt like being bitten by thousands of them from my thighs down to my toes. My legs literally felt like they were on fire. I screamed to the nursing assistant to lay me down immediately and requested ice to be put on my feet. The ice did not work but instead made it worse. My feet became really numb from the ice—a numbing effect that I have never felt before. I was grimacing in pain as I asked for my feet to be rubbed. The rubbing served as a distraction as the pain went from greater than level ten to level eight. Here I was thinking I had escaped the worst and was on the road to recovery, but I was about to discover the mystery pain. I remember a doctor entering the room and introducing herself as the neurologist. I wondered to myself, "Why do I need a neurologist?" She touched my legs, feet, and toes while asking about my level of sensation. To my dismay, I could not feel it when she touched certain areas on my legs or feet, but I experienced even more pain when she touched a particular part of my feet. I felt scared, angry, worried, and frustrated, among many other negative and frightening emotions.

I was told that I had developed peripheral neuropathy. I wanted to know what exactly caused it and how to fix it. This was not that easy, as my doctors also wanted to know what happened. I was given a medication called amitriptyline, which helped temporarily but caused rapid heartbeat. I would shift my head to look at the heart rate monitor and could see my heart beating in the 150s and hear the monitor alarms make their usual blaring sounds. The nurses would try to tell me to stay calm. Next, I was put on Neurontin, which was OK, except that it made me sleepy. At that time, though, I certainly preferred being sleepy to having a rapid heartbeat. I was told that I would need to take it until my pain went away or, by some chance of luck, my neuropathy went away.

At the end of October, I was transferred to an inpatient rehabilitation center, where I did physical therapy to learn how to walk with my inabilities. I was still on a regimen of ten to twelve tablets in the morning, and I had Coumadin injections, which I hated the most. They were just plain annoying, even though I know they were necessary to prevent blood clots. I did leg movements with my physical therapist and walked on a slow-moving treadmill while immersed in hip-deep water. This made it easier for me to walk and less the strain on my cardiovascular system. The pain I felt during this time was intense, and I can recall a few times not being the best patient. I was eating on my own, but I was constantly observed so I did not choke on my food. I was fed five times a day because by the time I was admitted to the rehab center, I had dropped to only 129 pounds. I am six feet tall, so

I was grossly underweight, and my nutrition needs were a top priority also. This was a difficult process, but I had the support of family and friends, which was a great encouragement.

Upon release from the rehab center in December 1998, I started regular visits to my neurologist. My pain from the neuropathy increasingly got worse, so my neurologist kept on upping the dosage. One day I took two doses too close to each other. I forgot that I had taken the first dose and took the other one. I was speaking to a friend on the phone and literally passed out.

Bony calcifications had formed in my hips—another complication that developed during my illness—and I had to have corrective hip surgery. My left foot was pointed permanently to the outside, and I had developed a foot drop (a condition where the foot points down because of weakened frontal leg muscles or tight calf muscles). I was afraid to have the surgery to correct it, fearing it would make my neuropathy worse. However, if I wanted to walk better and not trip all the time, surgery was necessary. Because the hip condition was so painful, it was necessary to take strong pain relievers, which made me very drowsy. I felt like life was piling all this on me. I was only twenty-five years old, and my life had changed drastically. My carefree life had turned into a life where I had disabilities and had to pay attention to how I conducted even simple activities of life. I would spend the next fourteen months going to physical therapy and then to a wellness center where I was taught exercises that were safe for me to perform.

My neurology visits continued. I was taking 900 mg of Neurontin three times daily. My body had gotten used to the dosage, so it was less sedating, but my pain was not decreasing. My neurologist wanted to increase the dosage once more, but I declined. I realized that I needed to keep a note or journal of how I felt when I woke up and during regular activities like taking a shower, eating, or going to physical therapy. If I could not fight peripheral neuropathy, I would have to learn to coexist with it and know the high and low points throughout each day, week, and month. I started reading medical journals and spoke to my primary physician and neurologists about what I was thinking. I wanted to have the pain gone or at least diminished so that I could live a life where I could go out with family and friends and not be confined at home curled up in pain. Over the next six months, I had a nerve biopsy, an electromyogram (EMG), and multiple appointments to find out more about my peripheral neuropathy. The nerve biopsy did not reveal much, except that there was damage caused perhaps by a huge inflammatory response during my illness. I was frustrated by the process not yielding as many answers as I wanted, given that I did so many tests and visited the neurologists so often.

I ventured out into the world of self-discovery with my peripheral neuropathy and started on my journey to find out as much as I could about the condition, since I was told it was permanent.

I started to analyze myself from the time I got up and throughout the day. I involved family and friends in this process to form a support system. Another reason that I involved family and friends is that most of the time, they felt helpless and didn't know how to really support me with my neuropathy. I asked my family and friends to observe me doing simple tasks at home, such as preparing meals and walking about, and to take note of what they observed about my level of fatigue, complaints about pain, and so forth.

I want you to note the following each morning immediately after you wake up:

1. How are you feeling?
2. Do you feel happy to be alive?
3. Are you excited to get the day going?
4. Do you have a purpose and a plan?
5. Are your feet numb, burning, aching, or tingling?
6. How do your hands feel?
7. How does your body feel?

Continue to assess how you feel throughout the day.

Two

Design Your Life

Designing your life is important to overcoming peripheral neuropathy. Having a design in place helps you to respond whenever you experience flare-ups. Yes, I have an occasional flare-up if I am not consistent with my plan. If I have had a few strenuous days where I don't sleep enough, forget to take my vitamins and supplements, and do not follow through with other parts of the plan, then I will receive a surprise in my feet. It is usually a sharp, shooting pain that exits through all my toes, and it can last anywhere from one to two minutes. This is noticeable by others, as it normally stops me abruptly in my tracks.

There are a few definitions for the word "design." I found these on www.dictionary.com, and they fit well: "An intention, purpose, end. An adaptation of means to a preconceived end."

In the beginning stages of my peripheral neuropathy, I would get up out of bed, get upset at stumbling because my feet were numb and hips ached, be upset at taking medication every few hours for the pain, and fighting with the pain. The list does not stop here. I have spoken to others with peripheral neuropathy and chronic pain and have heard similar stories. This went on for years. My mind was reacting to everything, and I was on constant high alert. I remember when things started to change. I was growing concerned about taking 900 mg of Neurontin three times daily and 500 mg of Vicodin once or twice daily and started looking for alternative methods. I was going to the gym often to keep my body (especially my legs) strong so I could continue to walk without the need of a walker or cane. My legs suffered the most as a result of peripheral neuropathy. I realized that I was not as strong as I was before. My grip was weak and my biceps were not as hard, even when I flexed. I noticed my other muscles were not as they were before. Therefore, I would need to constantly stimulate them.

So after stumbling one too many times, I decided to take precautionary measures and implemented my routine for the day. Here is an example of a typical day for me.

Upon Waking

1. I lie still and become aware of my body (one to two minutes). I visualize being at my favorite place by the ocean and listening to the waves, finding my center and feeling good.
2. I flex and point my toes ten times.
3. I tense and relax the muscles in my legs ten times.
4. I tense and relax my abdominal muscles five times, but I hold each time for around five seconds.
5. I tense and relax my arms ten times.
6. I slowly move my head from side to side four times.
7. I assess how my body feels after steps two through six.
8. I get up slowly and say thanks for being alive one more day.
9. I read, pray, and do the exercises planned for that day.
10. I drink one glass of water.
11. I take a shower.
12. I check my feet for any unusual bruises or cuts. (This is especially important if you have numbness in your feet or if you suffer from diabetic peripheral neuropathy.)
13. I get dressed for work.
14. I normally eat a banana and four ounces of juice for the ride to work.

During the Late Morning and Day

1. I eat an egg-white sandwich on whole wheat toast with orange or coconut juice. I take my vitamins and supplements after I eat. If you are tea or coffee drinker, you can have your morning cup.
2. I eat fruits, nuts (almonds, pistachios), or a fruit smoothie for snacks.
3. I drink around six to eight ounces of water each hour. My goal is to drink half my body weight in ounces of water and other decaffeinated beverages daily.
4. Lunch is usually chicken, beef, or fish with rice, beans, and vegetables. I use my lunch time to have fun, de-stress, or have meaningful conversations with others.
5. Dinner is normally in the late evening, with meat and a small portion of carbohydrates (rice, preferably brown, sweet potato, or pasta). I take my vitamins and supplements with dinner.
6. I spend time with my son and wife.
7. I do tasks such as answering questions regarding peripheral neuropathy from my website (http://www.LivingWithPeripheralNeuropathy.com or posting comments on my fan page (https://Facebook.com/Overcomingneuropathy checking and answering e-mail. I also set up coaching calls in the evenings.

Before Bed

1. I make a list of the things I plan to do the next day.
2. I reflect on the day and the things for which I am grateful.
3. I drink a glass of water and decompress.
4. I massage my feet gently.
5. I put on socks.
6. I drift off to sleep and try to get between seven and eight hours of sleep each night.

You can design your life to be in alignment with your passions and around your neuropathy. Know what your limits are—what you can and cannot do. Go for it and have fun. Don't allow your neuropathy to take away your joy. There is so much you can do. I made a bucket list of the things I wanted to do that I knew I was physically capable of doing. I am not advising you to do what is uncomfortable and irresponsible, but have fun. Design fun times in your life.

1. I wanted to go skydiving, so I informed my doctor what I had in mind. My heart was in great shape. I ensured I dressed appropriately in comfortable, formfitting, warm clothing and on landing, kept my feet up. I had a great time.
2. I was a passenger in a drag-racing experience. It can be dangerous, but I chose to do it. All the safety precautions were followed. I was with professionals and dressed in appropriate safety gear.
3. I go for nature walks or hikes. If you hike, choose an area that is mostly flat and not as challenging to start. I do this in the summer and warmer months as much as possible. In the colder months, as long as it is above 40 degrees, I dress warmly and go for a twenty-minute walk outside. This is good for the mind and body. And, of course, always get clearance from your doctor before starting any exercise activity.
4. I love to dance to Latin music and reggae.

There are many different activities, such as:

1. Bowling
2. Tennis
3. Volleyball
4. Badminton
5. Playing cards
6. Bingo

7. Scrabble
8. Chess
9. Pool
10. Swimming
11. Water aerobics and weight training
12. Chair exercises

Whatever activities you loved to do, assess with your physician if you can still do them or need to modify the way they are done. I was under the watchful eye of physical therapists, exercise physiologists, and personal trainers for three years after being released from the hospital to ensure that I used the correct form while doing exercises.

Is there something you have wanted to do? If so, discuss with your spouse, family member, or friend, or hire a life coach and explore the possibilities.

Designing a life that you have always dreamed of and including your peripheral neuropathy is the best recommendation I have. Before reading the next chapter, write down some goals that you have not achieved yet.

Three

Mind-set and Transmutation

Before you start or do anything, you need to have the correct mind-set. Overcoming peripheral neuropathy is a mind, body, and soul process. You need to have an open mind to learn and try something new. If you don't have an open mind and the willingness to experience something new, then you may miss what I am writing in this e-book. I had to go into unfamiliar territory and trust that I had it within myself to live a fulfilled life, even with my inabilities and the pain. You purchased the e-book, so you are already halfway there.

Let me define mind-set and transmutation:

Mind-set: A fixed mental attitude or disposition that predetermines a person's responses to and interpretations of situations. (www.thefreedictionary.com)

Transmutation: Change into another nature, substance, form, or condition (www.dictionary.com)

Mind-set

I had to adjust my mind-set regarding my illness and the conditions I now had to face. Life presents many challenges, and peripheral neuropathy is a big one. I developed the mind-set that I was going to find a way to overcome peripheral neuropathy and the pain associated with it. That was my principal goal. I knew that if I had the correct mind-set then my life would be different. I wanted to get to the point where I could wean off the medications I was taking and feel more in control of my life. *Let me just say and emphasize that there is absolutely nothing wrong with needing to take your medications to relieve your neuropathic pain, and you should always work closely with your neurologist regarding your medications.* I tried several medications and had varying degrees of side effects from them all. I discussed with my physician about weaning off my medications because I felt it was the right choice for me at the time. I remember when I started working full time in 2002 and the times I would be close to passing out on the train from the sedating medications I had taken. I could barely keep my eyes open at times. I could see people staring at me, but I could not even care at the moment what they thought of me. I was the one sitting there fighting to stay conscious and get to work. I am thankful that the ride to work was sometimes close to two hours so I was able to function when I arrived at work. I can now see where my caffeine dependence came from.

I had taken medications for my peripheral neuropathy and hip pain for five years. It was not easy, and at times I needed to take Vicodin for the pain in my hips. Nevertheless, I held on to the faith and hope that one day it would be possible for me to come off my medications. The more I believed in myself, the more enthusiastic I was about life. I was less depressed and I found myself going out more and taking walks. I became outward focused and less focused on what was happening on the inside. I started interacting with more people at work and church. The pain was still there, but I was trying to find a better way to deal with it.

Where are you with your mind-set? You can start *today* and decide that you are going to learn to overcome the pain and frustration. Yes, it is a decision that you must consciously make every morning until it becomes unconscious. The major hurdle begins in your mind, and if you can overcome this, you are halfway there to reducing the pain. You may find it difficult in the beginning, but keep on practicing. Remember your goal, and focus on the things that make you feel happy.

The Power of the Subconscious Mind

Look at your life. Are you living the life you want…on your terms? Are you happy with what you've created, or do you think it could be better? It is not impossible! You can do it! You must believe in your subconscious mind and know that it can allow you to lead a life of joy, less pain, and success.

Let's start off with a simple procedure. Use your subconscious mind as a way to get a good night's rest. Before going to bed at night, tell it affirmations. For example, "I am feeling better, and I am relaxed." Believe, focus on the words, and feel good.

Also, it's very important to think positively. Do not say to yourself, "I'm just never lucky," or "I'm just meant to be pain." Think the opposite: "I am lucky," or "Things always work out in my favor." If you have trouble believing yourself when you say them, then change them to become more believable. You can start small or say, "I am becoming pain-free."

Be still and listen to your subconscious mind. Close your eyes if need be, and do not force anything to come to you, but just be still and wait. I remember when I was not able to put the covers over my feet or even wear socks because of the pain. I had to literally look at my feet, know that they were there, and tell myself that the sheet does not hurt. I recalled the many times before peripheral neuropathy entered my life going to bed with the sheets over my feet. Each night I visualized and remembered that. I also gave myself a light massage, as my feet were extremely sensitive and would burn if anything touched them. I began doing an exercise by taking a light sheet and using it to partially cover my feet. I would use my mind to diffuse the pain up my leg, and I would focus on my feet and be OK with the sheet covering them. After a few weeks of doing this, and with the help of Neurontin, I was able to finally sleep with the sheets over my feet. This was a welcome victory for me, especially during the winter months. I used this technique with wearing socks, wearing my sneakers, and finally transitioning to dress shoes.

Transmutation

I discovered the term *transmutation* during my research. It reminded me of a lesson that I learned in physics class—that energy cannot be destroyed, but can be changed in its form. At this moment I decided I would not grit my teeth and fight the pain. I would learn to use the neuropathic pain as a source of energy in my life.

I used this technique during the times I wanted to give up. Exercise was a crucial part of my recovery, but the neuropathy and calcification in my hips made it hard. I felt pain during workouts, but I would use the power of transmutation to harness that pain and use it as energy to push onward. In the beginning, my workouts were under the watchful eye of a physical therapist or exercise physiologist. I learned that if I was not able to transmute the pain into energy for my workout, I needed to stop and rest.

I remember one day when I needed to walk to the train station because the bus I was supposed to take did not come as scheduled. The distance was about two miles, and from walking on the treadmill I knew it would take me close to an hour to complete the trip. As I started my journey, I began feeling slight pain in my left foot that is affected by my foot drop. I diverted the pain through visualization and kept walking. You can do this after getting to know your body and the different types of pain you feel. The learning is continuous. Halfway to the train station, I felt a really sharp pain that stopped me in my tracks. I sat down, flexed my feet, and checked to ensure there were not any cuts and continued to walk. I started off slowly, and I focused on the area of the pain and visualized in my mind arriving at the destination. I took slow, deliberate steps and focused on where I was going. I no longer felt the pain. I was able to walk a little faster, and I made my train.

Four

Nutrition

Over the years of living with peripheral neuropathy, one of the things that I have discovered is the crucial role that healthy eating and good nutrition played in how I felt. I have had times in my life where I was totally gung ho in terms of healthy eating and nutrition. I was juicing fresh fruits and vegetables and clung to a Mediterranean-style diet high in fruits, vegetables, and fish. On the flip side, I have also had longer periods where I didn't really watch what I ate. Mind you, I was never terribly overweight, but to be honest, I could probably stand to lose a few pounds. I didn't pay attention to the refined, processed foods that I consumed. In reality, my diet probably wasn't that different from the average American, but then again, the average American doesn't have to deal with neuropathy day in and day out. If I wanted to have the best possible quality of life, I knew that I had to make a change. I started to research the foods that are most helpful in neuropathy and the ones to avoid.

B Vitamins

One of the key nutrients that I discovered is the role of B complex vitamins. Thiamine (B_1), for example, is very important for a functioning nervous system. Thiamine deficiency is pretty rare, but is often seen in people who suffer from alcoholism. Alcohol actually interferes with thiamine absorption in the gut, which is one of the reasons it is so toxic to nerves. Therefore, limiting alcohol intake is very important to prevent worsening of neuropathy symptoms. Thiamine is found in whole grains, red meat, egg yolks, brown rice, berries, nuts, and green leafy vegetables.

Riboflavin (Vitamin B_2) is also important in maintaining a healthy nervous system. It helps to convert niacin and vitamin B_6 into their active forms so that they can be used effectively by the body. It is readily found in things such as whole grains, meats, eggs, and cheese.

Niacin (B_3) and pyridoxine (B_6) are also important in maintaining healthy nerves. Niacin is found in meats, fish, milk, eggs, legumes, and peanuts. Pyridoxine can be found in organ meats such as liver, as well as fish, brown rice, and whole-grain cereals.

Cyanocobalamin (Vitamin B_{12}) is crucial for forming and maintaining myelin, which protects our nerves. Myelin is the protective covering that surrounds our nerves and allows for proper nerve conduction. Think of it like the outer covering protecting wires. Without a covering, wires can get frayed and damaged. Myelin functions in a similar manner. Without it, our nerves won't function properly and we will have nerve damage. Consuming alcohol in large quantities can affect and decrease our body's ability to absorb this crucial nerve vitamin as well. Some good sources of vitamin B_{12} include liver, meats, egg yolks, poultry, and milk. I recommend taking the methylcobalamin form of vitamin B_{12}, as it is better absorbed than other forms of B_{12} such as cyanocobalamin.

Folic acid (vitamin B_9) interacts and works with vitamin B_{12} to make DNA and is important to all cells (including nerve cells) in the body and supports healthy nerve function. This is another vitamin decreased by excessive alcohol use. It is so important to the nervous system that pregnant woman are recommended to take folic acid supplements to reduce the risk of neural tube defects. Folic acid is found in liver, green vegetables, and whole-grain cereals.

Omega Fatty Acids

A good balance of omega 3 and omega 6 fatty acids is important in a healthy diet to help the nervous system. The typical American diet has about fourteen to twenty-five times more omega 6 fatty acids than omega 3 fatty acids, and this imbalance can cause health problems. A good omega 6 fatty acid to consume is linoleic acid, which can reduce inflammation in the body. Foods rich in linoleic acid are plant-based oils such as olive oil, sesame oil, pine nuts, flax, sunflower seeds, and pumpkin seeds. Studies have shown that taking linoleic acid for six months or more may reduce the symptoms of nerve pain in people with diabetic neuropathy.

Omega 3 fatty acids also play a key role in nerve health, and several studies have indicated that they may help prevent or even help treat certain peripheral nerve damage. One study published in the *Clinical Journal of Pain* had five neuropathic patients treated with high doses of omega 3 fish oils and found clinically significant pain reduction and improved function. One of the biggest sources of omega 3 fatty acids is fish. Salmon contains about 1200 to 2400 mg of omega 3s. Anchovies, blue fin tuna, sardines, and trout also contain a considerable amount of omega 3s. Shellfish such as shrimp and lobster contain about 100 to 200 mg.

There are other sources of omega 3s besides fish, for example, flaxseed and soybean oil. They can also be found in kidney and pinto beans, spinach, broccoli, and cauliflower.

Things to Avoid

Diabetes is one of the leading causes of peripheral neuropathy. Prolonged exposure to high blood sugar can damage your nerves and interferes with the ability of your nerves to transmit signals. For this reason, adhering to a careful diabetic diet and making sure your blood sugars are well controlled is important for maintaining the health of your nerves. Uncontrolled diabetes will actually worsen your neuropathic symptoms, and it is important to avoid this.

In addition, as was previously discussed, it is important to avoid excessive alcohol use. Excessive alcohol consumption inhibits the absorption of several important B vitamins that are essential to nerve health, leading to deficiencies and worsening of neuropathic symptoms.

For some people who are sensitive to gluten, this can be another cause of worsening neuropathic symptoms. Gluten sensitivity is an inherited condition that leads to an inflammatory, autoimmune response when gluten (which is the protein found in wheat, rye, barley, and some oats) is ingested. Some studies have linked certain causes of neuropathy with untreated gluten sensitivity. It may be beneficial to discuss with your doctor possibly getting tested for gluten sensitivity to see if this is something that should be avoided.

Another thing to try to minimize is refined, processed grains. Provided that there is no gluten sensitivity, whole grains are generally good to eat. When possible, it is best to substitute healthier whole-grain options instead of refined grains such as white rice, white bread, or white pasta. During the refining process, much of the fiber and B vitamins are removed from the grain. The part of the grain that is left is typically made of starchy carbohydrates that have little nutritional value left. Some of those nutrients and vitamins are added back during manufacturing, but are really just a fraction of what was removed in the first place. For this reason, whole grains are a better and healthier option.

Diet I Found Helpful

I have found that a Mediterranean-style diet emphasizes a lot of the recommended foods important for good nerve health and minimizes the things that don't. The typical Mediterranean diet includes the following:

1. Fish and eggs about three to four times per week
2. A high intake of virgin olive oil, fruits, nuts, and vegetables
3. Dairy in the form of milk, cheese, and yogurt

4. A moderate amount of meat and naturally saturated fats
5. Whole grains instead of refined white grains (white bread, white pasta, etc.)

A glass of wine is also a part of a typical Mediterranean diet, but I would try to limit that based on what we know about the potential effect alcohol can have on the nerves.

Overall, however, with the typical Mediterranean-style diet, you automatically consume high sources of omega 3s from the fish; a high amount of linoleic acid from the olive oil; and multiple B complex vitamins from whole grains, meats, eggs, and cheese. All of the aforementioned are important for maintaining healthy nerves.

In addition, I juice three to four times each week and make smoothies the other days. This is a great way for me to get in extra servings of fresh fruits and vegetables. I make green, red, orange, yellow, and purple juices. My favorite juice to make is green juice. It provides energy and is very nutritious. The ingredients are:

- 1 cup spinach
- 1 cup kale
- 1 small lime or lemon
- 2 green apples
- 1 small piece of ginger

My smoothie is usually made of:

- 1½ cups almond milk
- ½ cup oatmeal
- 1 banana
- 1 tablespoon honey
- 1 tablespoon almond butter (you can substitute peanut butter if preferred)

You can also find a seven-day meal plan for purchase at http://lwpnonline.com/meal-plan

Five

Exercise and Massage

Many types of exercises are available that can help you regain some of the strength that was lost due to peripheral neuropathy. Exercise was instrumental in helping me regain my independence and walk on my own. In the beginning, I had to regain my range of motion. I had severe restriction in my hips, and I had the foot drop on the left foot. I was very weak, especially in my legs, when I arrived at the inpatient rehabilitation facility. It was a humbling experiencing for me at twenty-five years old to be learning how to walk again and do the simple things in life like brushing my teeth, taking a shower, getting dressed, and feeding myself. I knew it was a long road, and I was feeling overwhelmed. The key to overcoming all of the doubts and anxiety was my mind-set, knowing my goals, and focusing on the present. I believed I would walk, become strong, and be able to do many of the things I used to do before.

During my rehabilitation, I asked what exercises would be used for me to regain my strength. My physician had prescribed what I could do based on my current situation. How familiar are you with exercise? Have you never exercised before? *Speak with your doctor to find out what you can and cannot do.* With peripheral neuropathy, your muscles don't receive the normal signals from the brain as before. How severe this is depends on the type of neuropathy you have and where your body is affected. Exercise increases your strength, flexibility, balance, stamina, and mood and can help you maintain or lose weight. It has also been shown to improve sleep and one's outlook on life. It is fun, too, if you do it with a family member or friend. You can go for a leisurely walk and have a conversation while walking about current events or your topic of choice. Exercise can help you too even if you are not that mobile. There are many different exercises, ranging from weight-bearing exercises to build muscle strength and yoga. They are countless cardiovascular exercises, such as using elliptical machines, swimming, walking, cycling, jogging, aqua aerobics, tennis, badminton, golf, and dancing. You can also do different chair exercises. Do not attempt jogging, tennis, badminton, cycling, or complex dancing (quick turns and other challenging moves that require balance) if your balance is impaired. You can combine weight training and cardiovascular training on the same or separate days. *It cannot be said enough: Always consult your physician before starting an exercise program.*

The Benefits of Various Types of Exercise

Weight Training or Weight Bearing

The main benefit of weight training is that it strengthens your bones and helps to prevent osteoporosis. For adults who already have weak or thinning bones, take it slowly and be consistent. Do not lift heavy weights. Weight training also builds muscle strength. Strong muscles help to keep you stable and increase your balance. You should consider getting an introductory session with a personal trainer at any gym you join. I joined a wellness center, even though I exercised often before my illness and peripheral neuropathy. I wanted to ensure I would not injure myself while I was exercising, as my body was not the same as before. You can do exercises at home without weights if you are not able to join a gym, but you should have someone in the home with you in the beginning.

I will list the exercises I did for weight training and continue to do today. I exercised my entire body even though my lower body needed more attention. The exercises are:

Lower Body

- Leg press
- Leg extension
- Leg curl
- Standing or seated calf raise
- Hip abductor and adductor exercise
- Toe raise

Upper Body

- Seated machine back row
- Lateral pull-down to the front of chest
- Seated machine incline chest press
- Seated machine chest press
- Seated machine shoulder press
- Front and side lateral raise for shoulders
- Machine biceps curls
- Machine triceps extension
- Triceps dips (with supervision)
- Machine forearm curls

The machine exercises were recommended in the beginning because I needed more stability and controlled movement. Free weights were used at times for the shoulder press, raises, and biceps and triceps curls, but at a low weight that did not exceed five pounds. As I became stronger, the amount was increased. I did one to three sets of ten repetitions of each exercise, depending on how I felt physically that day. You should engage your mind with your body as you exercise to get the full benefits. Pay attention to the movement you are doing.

At home, I do the following:

- Wall squats
- Standing calf raise
- Pushups on hands and knees

Cardiovascular Exercises

Cardiovascular exercise has many benefits:

- Improved heart and lung health
- Improved endurance
- Stress relief
- Improved mood
- Lower blood pressure
- Better oxygen delivery to the cells of the body (just as sleep is important to rejuvenate the body, your nerves need oxygen-rich blood)

There are many different recommendations for cardio exercises, from thirty minutes three to five days a week to seven days a week. Do an activity that elevates the heart rate from the previous list, such as light to brisk walking or your favorite activity or exercise. However, you should do the amount depending on your current state as assessed by your physician.

I started with walking outdoors along with using a stationary bike and the elliptical machine. Walking outdoors and the elliptical machine are two of my favorite exercises. I would use the treadmill whenever walking outdoors was not possible. You can choose your favorite exercise that is safe for you to do.

Walking Outdoors

Walking outdoors in the park, around a track, or around your neighborhood streets has many advantages:

1. You are outside breathing fresh air.
2. The environment changes, depending on where you walk.
3. You interact with other people.
4. You get vitamin D from the sunlight and it elevates your mood.

I vary my routine to eliminate boredom. I walk in my neighborhood fifteen to twenty minutes in one direction, then I turn around and walk the same distance back home. At times, I go to the park and walk around the pond for thirty minutes. Doing nature walks with my wife and son has become one of my favorites. You can invite family or friends to walk with you. Ensure that you wear reflective clothing or sneakers if you like to walk in the early morning or late evening, and walk facing the traffic if possible if there is no sidewalk.

Stationary Bike

Stationary bikes are great for those who enjoy cycling but are unable to do so safely. I love doing this exercise and normally ride for thirty minutes whenever I do. During my recovery, I used the stationary bike at least once or twice weekly. Be careful when dismounting from the stationary bike if you are prone to your feet becoming numb.

Elliptical Machine

I remember when I first used the elliptical machine. It was like effortless running. However, after adjusting the settings, I realized that it could be as challenging as the stair climber but easier to do. I was a big stair climber fan, and I loved to run. When I was a kid, I ran everywhere, often preferring running instead of walking. However, after my hospitalization, running and using the stair climber were decreased. I don't run anymore because of my left foot drop, and I seldom use the stair climber.

One surprising benefit of the elliptical machine in combination with the weight training is that it helped me regain some of the balance that I had lost on my left side. Always hold onto the handles while using the elliptical if you don't have good balance. Even if your balance is great, it is still good practice to hold onto the handles. The elliptical has become the most used cardiovascular activity for me, as it satisfies my love for running that I miss so much.

Massage

The holistic application of physical touch to affect the systems of the body is called a body massage. Therapeutic massage originated in China and is an age-old healing art that can alleviate mental, physical, and emotional ailments.

Body massage helps release stress and tension in our bodies by increasing oxygen flow and blood circulation. Excessive unresolved tension and stress in our daily lives could cause continuous muscular tension. This type of mental tension or stress diminishes the flow of oxygen and blood to the muscles and organs, causing pains and aches, feelings of fatigue, symptomatic heaviness, tightness of muscles, and stiffness. This can even increase the chance of strains and injuries. Tension creates a tendency for a buildup of toxins in the body and reduces the flow of the more subtle energy or life force (prana or chi). Muscular stress also deforms the skeletal anatomy, which further compounds present problems and develops new ones.

Benefits of Body Massage

1. Assists weight loss
2. Improves and increases blood circulation and the flow of tissue fluid (lymph)
3. Nourishes the skin with the right oils
4. Soothes and relaxes nerves

5. Assists in removal of deposits of tissue
6. Releases emotional and mental tension
7. Creates a feeling of well-being
8. Gives pleasure

If you have any illness, it is always advisable to inform a doctor before you go for a body massage.

Precautions

1. Wear appropriate clothing for the type of exercise you are doing and climate that you are in. Wear comfortable clothing like shorts, sweats, and sneakers. If you are going for a leisurely walk, then you don't you have to be in sportswear, but it is best to be in loose clothing and sneakers or other prescribed walking shoe.
2. Ask for help from the staff if you are in a gym and are unfamiliar with a form of exercise.
3. Be aware of your surroundings while exercising.
4. Be careful when you are finished doing cardio. Take care when getting off exercise equipment. With peripheral neuropathy, the numbness or balance issues can cause falls. I found out that my feet get numb if I stay on the cross-trainer, rowing machine, or stationary bike for more than five minutes.
5. Stop if you feel uncomfortable, are in pain, or have difficulty breathing.
6. Start slowly and don't overdo it.

Six

Spirituality, Meditation, and Yoga

Spirituality and meditation are pivotal to me. Most people believe in a higher power. Many pray, meditate, chant, and so forth. I personally pray to God and believe that He gives me what I need to function, no matter what the circumstance. Here I was for many years praying and believing, but my heart was not content. I was not joyful and I was not grateful. Yes, I was happy to be alive. I had survived an illness that not many people survive. I had spent two months in the intensive care unit (ICU) with my life hanging in the balance. I took an analysis of what was going on within my heart and mind. I was still hanging onto anger and bitterness for what had happened after so many years. I thought I had let go of all the negative emotions, but I was wrong. Hanging onto all these emotions, feeling wronged by the same God I believed in, was in the background and did not help me heal internally. This manifested in my body, and I experienced pain on a scale of eight to nine most of the days.

I decided I needed to release this negative energy. Overall, I needed to love who I was and had become as a result of my ordeal. Once I decided to do this, it was like a weight was lifted off my head. I felt lighter. I prayed for the strength to continue to love myself, for acceptance of what had happened, and to live with a purpose. I was no longer afraid of people knowing that I did not have a perfect body, that I had scars, that my feet did not work properly, that I had pain, and that I felt depressed and angry most times. I could talk about what had happened to me without fear. I was able to love through the anger I felt. I forgave myself.

Meditation

Here's the Mayo Clinic's viewpoint on the benefits of meditation:
"Meditation is used by people who are perfectly healthy as a means of stress reduction. But if you have a medical condition that's worsened by stress, you might find the practice valuable in reducing the stress-related effects of allergies, asthma, chronic pain, and arthritis, among others."

Benefits of Meditation

Among the documented benefits of meditation are less anxiety; decreased depression; reduction in irritability and moodiness; and improvements in learning ability, memory, and creativity. That's just for starters. Then there is slower aging, feelings of vitality and rejuvenation, less stress, lower metabolic and heart rate, lower blood pressure, and higher blood oxygen levels.

How to Meditate Right Now

Breathe, and watch your breath.
Here's a simple technique that will give you results in minutes. Sit comfortably, close your eyes, and tense up your whole body. Sigh deeply, then breathe deeply through your nose and release the tension from every muscle. Just feel each part relaxing, watching for parts that may hold onto tension, like a tight jaw.
If you still have tension somewhere, tense up that part again, then let it relax. It may also help to repeat silently the word

"relax" as the tension drains. This will train your body and mind to recognize relaxation. Later, you may be able to relax more easily just by repeating "relax" a few times.

Breathe through your nose. This is important because it brings in more oxygen by involving your diaphragm more. You can test this. Breathe with your mouth and you'll notice that your breathing is shallower. Then breathe through your nose and you'll notice that your abdomen extends more. Air is being drawn deeper into your lungs.

Allow your breathing to fall into a comfortable pattern, and pay attention to it. Pay attention to your breath as it passes in and out of your nose. Your mind may wander endlessly, but all you have to do is continually bring attention back to your breath.

If your mind is still too busy, try naming the distractions as a way of setting them aside. For example, say in your mind, "itchy leg," "worried about work," or "anger," and then immediately return attention to your breathing. Use any method you can to identify and set aside distractions.

That's it. Continue for five or ten minutes, or for one hundred breaths. Afterward, open your eyes and sit there for a few seconds. You'll feel relaxed, and your mind will feel refreshed. And you'll be better prepared for any mental challenges. That is how to meditate.

You can find a free meditation guide here: http://lwpnonline.com/optin

Yoga

I discovered yoga in late 2003, and it was amazing. I was not as flexible as the others, my balance was not the greatest, but I believed I could do it. I informed the yogi leading the class of my inabilities, and his answer was the best. He said, "Yoga is about finding your center, your peace. It is your own personal journey, and you do what your body can do. Listen to your body and challenge yourself a little more each time, but never overdo it. Be OK with where you are, see where you want to go, and do it. Don't compare yourself to anyone else." Yoga gave me more than increased flexibility and balance. It also calmed my spirit, and this helped to calm my body.

The Benefits of Yoga

The practice of yoga brings with it many physical and emotional benefits that the majority of people are unaware of. Yoga is a science; indeed, in many places in the world (such as India), it is referred to as a science. Yoga as a science seeks to understand how the body acts and reacts to changes in the internal physical environment.

Yoga involves a series of postures, during which you pay special attention to your breathing—exhaling during certain movements and inhaling with others. You can approach yoga as a way to promote physical flexibility, strength, and endurance or as a way to enhance your spirituality.

The Mind-Body Connection

Yoga is centered on the mind-body connection. This harmony is achieved through three things:

- Postures (asanas)
- Proper breathing (pranayama)
- Meditation

Physical Benefits

By harmonizing these three principles, the benefits of yoga are attained. And just what are these benefits?

- Equilibrium in the body's central nervous systemDecrease in pulse, respiratory, and blood pressure rates
- Cardiovascular efficiency

- Gastrointestinal system stabilization
- Increased breath-holding time
- Improved dexterity
- Improved balance
- Improved depth perception
- Improved memory

Psychological Benefits

In addition, yoga delivers an array of psychological benefits; in fact, this is a common reason why people begin practicing it in the first place. Perhaps the most frequently mentioned psychological benefit of yoga is an improved ability to manage stress. Yoga diminishes an individual's levels of anxiety, depression, and lethargy, thus enabling you to focus on what's spiritual and important: achieving balance and happiness.

Seven

Dreams and Goals

It is never too late to dream and to have goals. Dreams and goals give us a reason to wake up, live our lives, and celebrate, whether it is a small or big victory. No matter what stage you are at in life, you can dream and you can fulfill that dream.

What is a dream? A dream is a goal, an aspiration, or aim (www.dictionary.com).

I remember having dreams of walking; being able to put the blanket over my feet; wearing my socks, sneakers, and dress shoes; getting married; becoming a parent; helping others with peripheral neuropathy and chronic pain; skydiving; driving in an exotic car (Lamborghini, Ferrari, Maserati); visiting other states in the United States; having fun; connecting with nature; and many more. The dreams did not happen overnight, but I wrote my dreams and goals down in a journal. I set target dates for achieving my dreams. I achieved some dreams by my set date, but others I missed. Don't feel bad about missing a target date—it is your dream and you can still achieve it. Keep your dream book close to you and look at your dreams daily, weekly, and monthly. Choose the dream that is most important to you and start with it first—think about it, see it already achieved in your *mind, believe it,* and do the action steps needed to achieve it. Your dreams should inspire you, and you should feel good about them in your mind. Feeling good is important in daily life and especially with peripheral neuropathy and pain. If you don't feel good in your mind, it is more difficult to feel good in your body. Share your dreams with a family member or close friend who supports you and ask to be kept accountable.

The Power of the Subconscious Mind

You can live the life you want. Think about the greatness you can achieve by using your entire mind. I'm here to tell you that you currently possess the most powerful tool in the universe—your *subconscious mind*. Your subconscious mind knows everything. It has all the answers if you just use it correctly. It can lead you to a life of harmony, health, joy, and success! This is possible with all aspects of your life.

The past is over, and today can be a new start. It doesn't matter what happened before today—what matters is what happens from today on. You must believe in your subconscious mind and know that it can allow you to lead a life of less pain, more joy, and more fulfillment.

The first step in changing your life is to start making impressions on your subconscious mind. You can do this by making affirmations, as well as thinking certain thoughts. For example, let's say you were thinking of going on your favorite vacation to Jamaica or Hawaii. You can simply repeat these words: "I am on the beach in Jamaica, and I feel great." Repeat these words several times a day. It's best to say them in the morning when you get up and right before you sleep when your mind is in a relaxed state. When saying them, make sure you really mean them and focus on the words. Try not to view it as a chore, or else it will not do you much good. You can also say your affirmations while meditating.

This can work for anything. Make sure the affirmations are positive and not stating the negative. For example, if you want to reduce your pain, don't say, "I don't want pain." Instead say, "My body is healthy, and I am pain-free." "I am" are two of the most powerful words in the English language. Think positively about your dreams.

I achieved most of the dreams noted earlier over the last fourteen years, and I have set new goals. Each day I think about the goal I am focused on and do an action to get closer to achieving it.

You can see me achieving one of my goals by clicking this link and looking at the photos. You will see me driving a Lamborghini. https://www.facebook.com/overcomingneuropathy

Write your goals down before going on to the next chapter and place a number from one to ten based on their importance to you (ten being the goal that is most important). Start working on the goals that are tens and work your way down. Goals that are sevens or sixes will move up as you achieve your other goals.

Get introductory coaching sessions that can help you attain your goals at http://lwpnonline.com/coaching.

Eight

Medication, Supplementation, and Devices

Various options are available, both conventional and alternative, in regard to treatment of peripheral neuropathy. Some of the more conventional treatments include medications or medical procedures such as plasmapheresis, transcutaneous electrical nerve stimulation/percutaneous electrical nerve stimulation (TENS/PENS), or surgery. In cases where peripheral neuropathy is caused by compression from a herniated disc, for example, surgical intervention can often reverse the symptoms of peripheral neuropathy. In addition to the already mentioned treatment options, several complementary supplements are available that may help improve the symptoms of peripheral neuropathy. These complementary supplements include things such as B complex vitamin supplements, fish and primrose oils, acupuncture, massage, and biofeedback.

Medications

There are several medications for neuropathy that can help treat its painful symptoms. Certain antidepressants within what is called the tricyclic family of medications can reduce burning, stabbing, aching, and throbbing sensations of peripheral neuropathy. Some of these medications include amitriptyline, nortriptyline, imipramine, and desipramine. Duloxetine is another antidepressant approved to manage neuropathic pain related to diabetes.

Some medications typically used in epilepsy can also be effective in reducing sharp and stabbing neuropathic pain. These drugs include Tegretol, Neurontin, Lyrica, Topamax, and Lamictal.

Topical anesthetics such as lidocaine creams or capsaicin creams can provide temporary relief for pain localized to one area. The previously mentioned antidepressant and antiepileptic medications are typically considered first-line treatment options for painful peripheral neuropathy. For severe pain, however, narcotics such as codeine, oxycodone, morphine, or fentanyl patches may be used if the first-line treatments are ineffective.

Plasmapheresis

Plasmapheresis is a procedure in which the blood is purified from circulating antibodies. It is essentially a process where antibodies are filtered out from the blood. First, a long tube known as a catheter is placed in a central vein. The blood is then removed from the body, and the blood cells are subsequently separated from the plasma. Plasma is the liquid part of blood in which antibodies are found. The blood cells are then returned back to the body, along with either fresh or substitute plasma. This procedure may be helpful if the peripheral neuropathy is caused by antibodies attacking the peripheral nerves, and if it is used quickly enough before permanent damage can occur. Filtering out these antibodies may alleviate some of the symptoms of peripheral neuropathy.

TENS/PENS

TENS and PENS can be helpful in alleviating some of the more painful symptoms of peripheral neuropathy, but have to be used repeatedly to sustain the benefits.

During TENS procedures, a small battery-operated device is worn by the patient, and electrodes are typically placed on the surface of the skin over the area where the pain is felt. A low-level electrical current is then applied for usually about thirty minutes, several times throughout the day.

The PENS procedure is similar in concept to TENS. The main difference is that instead of using the surface electrodes seen in TENS devices, PENS uses needle probes as electrodes that are inserted through the skin. These needle probes are typically placed next to the nerve causing painful neuropathy symptoms and then stimulated. PENS can be used in people who do not get sufficient pain relief from TENS.

Complementary Treatments

B Complex Vitamin Supplements

There are eight known B vitamins. These vitamins are all considered water soluble, meaning that any excess amounts are excreted in the urine. They are found in sources such as meat, beans, potatoes, and whole grains.

B complex vitamins are important for overall health and well-being, and many play an important role in healthy nerve function. B complex vitamin supplements may help to improve some mild to moderate symptoms of peripheral neuropathy. Vitamin B_{12} in particular plays a role in the formation and maintenance of myelin, which is the sheath covering surrounding the nerve. B_{12} is also available as a shot and can be given every few weeks to help with neuropathy symptoms if your neurologist recommends it. However, caution must be used with supplements because excessive amounts of B_6 and B_{12} vitamins can lead to peripheral neuropathy as well. Follow the recommended dosages, and always consult your physician before using any supplements.

Fish Oil and Evening Primrose Oil

Fish oils are known to be an excellent source of essential fatty acids. This is important in terms of peripheral neuropathy because about 80 percent of myelin is made up of fats. Docosahexaenoic acid (DHA), in particular, is one of the essential fatty acids that line the nervous system and is used for rapid message relay. When looking for these supplements, it is often best to look for ones that are high in DHA.

Evening primrose oil is a rich source of linoleic acid, which is further broken down into gamma-linolenic acid (GLA). GLA is another essential fatty acid that is important to the makeup of myelin. Clinical studies have shown that primrose oil supplements may help to improve nerve function and may help reduce some mild to moderate symptoms of peripheral neuropathy.

(You can get your supplements here if you shop on Amazon: http://amzn.to/1zNswpa.)

Acupuncture

Acupuncture typically involves inserting sterile needles into specific points in the body to stimulate the flow of chi, or vital energy. It is believed to work by stimulating the brain to release chemicals into the body that reduce sensitivity to pain and is also believed to activate nerve receptors that decrease pain signals. Needles are typically left in place for about thirty minutes while being stimulated either by twirling or by applying electrical stimulation to the needles. A small study published in the *European Journal of Neurology* found that 76 percent of patients who received acupuncture had improvement in their pain symptoms and had improved nerve conduction of the peripheral nerves.

Massage Therapy/Reflexology

Massage therapy can also be helpful in managing neuropathic pain and is very relaxing. One of the most common forms of massage used for neuropathy is Swedish massage. Massages can aid in pain relief, increase circulation to the area being massaged, and stimulate nerves. Massage can also release endorphins to help fight pain.

Reflexology is a form of massage that typically involves applying pressure to the feet, hands, or ears with specific thumb or hand pressure techniques. One study involving seventy-six patients found that after using reflexology techniques over the course of six weeks there was reduction in neuropathic symptoms, particularly tingling sensations and pain.

Biofeedback

Biofeedback may be helpful in reducing stress and coping with neuropathic pain. During a biofeedback session, electrical sensors are typically applied to different parts of your body, which allows for monitoring of your body's physiological responses such as heart rate and breathing in response to pain. Over time, you are able to monitor and learn to consciously manage your body's physiological responses using the feedback machine. You begin to recognize your body's responses to pain and you can learn ways to lessen that pain through certain techniques such as relaxation or guided imagery.

Nine

Live Your Life

So here we are on the last chapter. Congratulations on getting here. You have your whole life ahead of you. I know you have plans for vacations, outdoor adventures, trips to the museum, visits to the theater, and more. Go out and do what you love and enjoy.

Waking up each morning and being grateful for seeing another day is a big help. I had to make this change. Even before my peripheral neuropathy and inability to run or walk, I would get up some mornings in a bad mood, especially in the winter. I love the warm weather and the sun. Now I wake up feeling grateful to be alive one more day, even when it is raining and cold outside. Find ways to include something fun in your day. Remember the things you used to do before peripheral neuropathy or chronic pain and see if you are still able to do these tasks or activities.

Don't be afraid to reach out to family for help if needed. Sometimes it may be difficult to prepare a meal, clean, go for a walk, and do the simple things. Make the phone call to a family member or friend, or ask someone if you are living in the same home. I have done that at times and I have received the assistance I needed.

Here is a list of just ten things out of many you could do:

- Go for daily walks in the park.
- Have a game night with friends.

- Learn something new.
- Volunteer at a local hospital.
- Go to the museum.
- Visit family and friends.
- Read a book series or watch movies.
- Review your goals and dreams.
- Start a gratitude journal.
- Develop a new hobby—for example, writing.

Overall, remember to be grateful for each day and feel good. It does wonders for your mind, body, and soul.

(You can be a part of the Living with Peripheral Neuropathy membership area for only a penny for the first month: http://lwpnonline.com/thank-you.)

Frequently Asked Questions (FAQ)

What exactly is peripheral neuropathy?

Simply put, peripheral neuropathy is any disorder or condition that affects the peripheral nerves—that is, the nerves outside the brain and spinal cord.

How common is peripheral neuropathy?

Peripheral neuropathy is actually quite common. The prevalence is estimated to be about 3 percent to 8 percent of the general population and affects about twenty million people in the United States.

What are some of the common symptoms of peripheral neuropathy?

People can experience many different peripheral neuropathy symptoms. In the early stages, symptoms can come and go, and a physical exam may even be normal. Symptoms are typically classified as either sensory or motor in nature. Usually, the sensory symptoms would come first, with motor symptoms becoming more prominent as the neuropathy progresses.

Sensory symptoms refer to those symptoms that cause altered sensations. Paresthesia is a fancy term that is often used to describe any abnormal or unusual sensation that people with peripheral neuropathy experience. Some common paresthesias include pins and needles, burning, tingling, numbness, and shocklike sensations.

In many cases, these paresthesias have a "stocking-glove" distribution. The term "stocking-glove" means that the abnormal sensations often start in the toes and feet, work their way up to the knees, and then appear in the hands.

Some paresthesias cause people to feel pain from things not normally painful (for example, warm or cold water on the skin feels painful). Other people, especially diabetics, have decreased feeling and numbness in their feet. Regular foot checks are very important for these individuals because if they get a cut or an injury, they may not realize it.

Motor symptoms of peripheral neuropathy typically refer to the effects the neuropathy has on a person's movement. One of the common complaints of people with peripheral neuropathy is muscle weakness. The muscles surrounding the affected nerve may even start to waste away and appear smaller than usual. This occurs as a result of the muscles not being stimulated enough due to the damaged nerves that run through them. On physical examination, a person's reflexes may be decreased or absent. This is considered to be one of the measurable signs of peripheral neuropathy. This condition can affect the way a person walks, as well as their balance. Due to the decrease in balance, people with severe peripheral neuropathy are more prone to falls and injury. A person with peripheral neuropathy may take higher steps to prevent their toes from dragging and may slap their feet on the ground when walking.

What are some of the causes of peripheral neuropathy?

The potential peripheral neuropathy causes that have been identified are numerous and varied. In fact, many different diseases and illnesses can result in this potentially debilitating condition. At times, the resulting peripheral neuropathy is only temporary and can be reversed completely. This, of course, would really depend on the particular cause and whether or not it can be rectified with appropriate treatment. Other times, however, the symptoms of peripheral neuropathy can become permanent. Some of the more common illnesses or conditions that can cause it include nerve compression from a herniated disc in your back, diabetes, trauma, autoimmune illnesses, critical illnesses, nutritional deficiencies, HIV, or alcoholism.

What kind of tests or studies might my doctor do?

After taking a full medical, social, and family history, your doctor may want to start with some basic blood tests to make sure that you are not deficient in certain vitamins, which can be a cause of neuropathy. They may also want to get a computed tomography (CT) scan or magnetic resonance imaging (MRI) to look for any herniations that can cause neuropathy. They would likely do a neurological exam to check your reflexes and muscle strength.

In addition, your doctor may want to do more specialized studies. They may want to do a nerve biopsy where they take a small sample of your nerve to check for any abnormalities. They may want to do nerve conduction studies to see how well your nerves send and receive signal messages.

Are there any additional resources or support groups that may help me?

Here is a listing of some helpful resources. In addition, you can find a list of local support groups by going to the Neuropathy Association website listed here.

The Neuropathy Association
60 E. 42nd Street, Suite 942
New York, NY 10165
Phone: 212-692-0662
http://www.neuropathy.org

American Chronic Pain Association
PO Box 850
Rocklin, CA 95677
Phone: 1-800-533-3231
Fax: 916-632-3208
http://www.theacpa.org

Speaking with Me

If you want to set up personalized coaching sessions or have general questions, you can e-mail me at:
dlewis@livingwithperipheralneuropathy.com.

Please like my Facebook page at https://Facebook.com/OvercomingNeuropathy.

Other Links

These are links that were included in previous chapters for easy access.

Free meditation
http://lwpnonline.com/optin
Meal plan
http://lwpnonline.com/meal-plan
Membership area
http://lwpnonline.com/thank-you
Introductory coaching
http://lwpnonline.com/coaching

References and Resources

References

Ang, C. D., et al. "Vitamin B for treating peripheral neuropathy (review)." *The Cochrane Collaboration.* 2008, Issue 4.

Bauer, Joy. "Refined Grains: How Food Affects Health." www.joybauer.com/food-articles/refines-grains.aspx , January 12, 2014.

Beers, Mark, et al. *Merck Manual* (2nd ed.). Merck Research Laboratories, 2004.

"Diabetic Neuropathy." http://www.mayoclinic.org/diseases-conditions/diabetic-neuropathy/basics/causes , January 14, 2014.

"Emedicine." http://emedicine.medscape.com/article/325107-overview.

Fauci, A. S. and E. Braunwald, et al. *Harrison's Principles of Internal Medicine* (17th ed.). McGraw-Hill Companies, 2008.

Frontera, W. R., J. Silver, et al. *Essentials of Physical Medicine and Rehabilitation* (2nd ed.). Saunders, 2008

Goldman, Lee, et al. *Cecil's Textbook of Medicine* (23rd ed.). Elsevier Health Publishing, 2007.

Gordon, Jerry. "Ultimate Guide to B Vitamins." www.health.howstuffworks.com/wellness/food-nutrition/vitamin-supplements/vitamin-b.htm , January 9, 2014.

Gray, Nathan. Omega-3 fatty acids may prevent and treat nerve damage: Study http://mobile.nutraingredients.com/Research/Omega-3-fatty-acids-may-prevent-and-treat-nerve-damage-Study#.VKDKOF4AKA , January 9, 2014

Hadjivassiliou, M., R. A. Grunewald, et al. "Neuropathy Associated with Gluten sensitivity." *Journal Neurol Neurosurg Psychiatry* 77, no. 11 (November 2006): 1262–1266.

Halat, K. M., and C. E. Dennehy. "Botanicals and Dietary Supplements in Diabetic Peripheral Neuropathy." *The Journal of the American Board of Family Practice* 16 (2003): 47–57.

Hensle, Glenn. "Neurological (Nerve) Pain and Acupuncture." www.ezinearticles.com/?Neurological-(Nerve)-Pain-and-Acupunture&amp.com , January 15, 2014.

Jeong, I. S. "Effect of self foot reflexology on peripheral blood circulation and peripheral neuropathy in patients with diabetes mellitus." *Journal of Korean Acad Fundamental Nursing* 13, no. 2 (2006): 225–234.

Jones, Niya. "9 Diet Dos and Don'ts for Diabetic Neuropathy." www.inhealthcnn.com , January 16, 2014.

Ko, G. D., and N. B. Nowacki. "Omega 3 Fatty Acids for Neuropathic Pain: Case Series." *Clinical Journal of Pain* 26, no. 2 (February 2010): 168–172.

McLaughlin, August. "Foods That Fight Neuropathy." www.livestrong.com , January 16, 2014.

"Peripheral Neuropathy; Alternative Treatments." www.mayoclinic.com , January 15, 2014.

"Peripheral Neuropathy Diet and Treatment." www.livestrong.com , January 16, 2014.

Roycor, Alberto. "What Is the Mediterranean Diet?" www.mediterraneandiet.com , January 9, 2104.

Schroder, S., and J. Liepert. "Acupuncture treatment improves nerve conduction in peripheral neuropathy." *Eur J Neurol* 14, no. 3 (March 2007): 276–281.

Resources

You can purchase your supplements at your favorite online store—for example, Amazon (http://amzn.to/1zNswpa), a local pharmacy, or supplement store. Always inform your doctor of any supplements that you take.

These are tips and affirmations I wish I had when I first discovered I had peripheral neuropathy. They may seem small and insignificant, but they helped me tremendously over the years in other areas of my life also. Peripheral Neuropathy: Daily Tips and Affirmations: http://amzn.to/1vRuuG9.

Printed in Great Britain
by Amazon